To health

Copyright © 2017 Jason Drysdale

All rights reserved.

ISBN-13: 978-1497510258
ISBN-10: 1497510252

5th Edition

# One Meal A Day

Jason A. Drysdale

"A person who won't read has no advantage over one who can't read." – Mark Twain

# CONTENTS

**Chapter 1** ..............................................7
The origin of one meal a day

**Chapter 2** ..............................................11
Why one meal a day

**Chapter 3** ..............................................13
The benefits of one meal a day

**Chapter 4** ..............................................17
Getting started

## BONUS SECTION

**Olive oil secrets** ...................................21

**The truth about salt** ............................27

**Supreme health** ...................................33

"It is health that is real wealth and not pieces of gold and silver." — Mahatma Gandhi

# The Origin of One Meal a Day

I first came across the concept of one meal a day in the book; **How to Eat to Live** by Elijah Muhammad. In that book he mentioned that he learned the knowledge of one meal a day from W.D. Fard.

The one meal per day concept has been around for thousands of years, it is nothing new. Our ancient ancestors from the east used it for health and to live a long time. This is the secret that the ancients have used in order to live for hundreds of years.

The ancient people lived a very long time on our planet. Many lived to two hundred, three hundred, five hundred, and even much more. Methuselah lived to be nine hundred and sixty nine years old. A matter of fact; man can live as long as he choose to live, but he must first know how to eat to live in order to extend life. It starts with one meal per day. That's the very basic, minimum level.

If you want to extend your life even more than one hundred and twenty years, one meal every two days could extend your life to approximately one hundred and forty years old. One meal every three days can extend your life to one hundred and sixty years old, and it goes on up to one meal every seven days.

This is the way of our forefathers which has been kept secret for many years. All you need to know is the proper way of eating one meal a day and then you'll realize that it's not impossible and that it is quite easy.

If you think that this is a bit farfetched, then consider this: If bowhead whales can live for hundreds of years, then what about man?

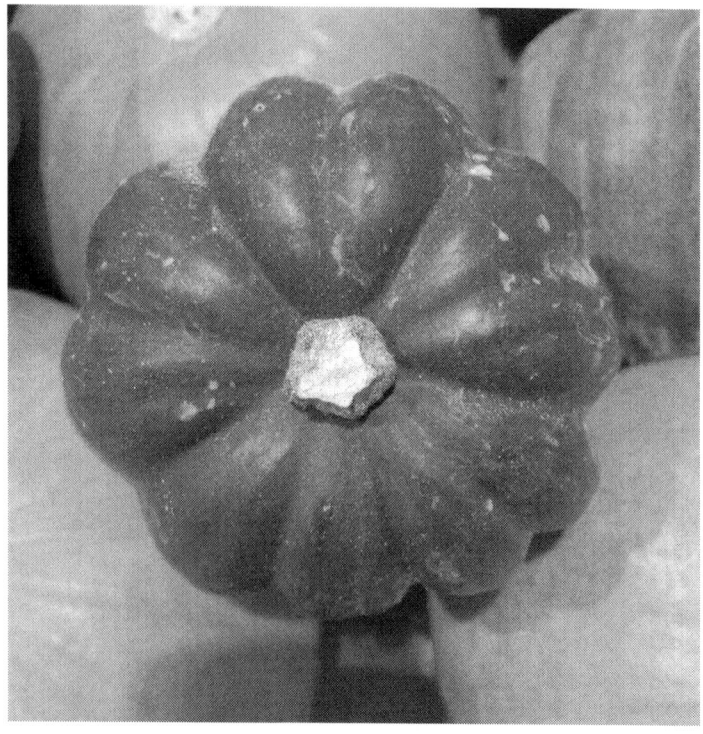

Man is the best and brightest creation, with unlimited potential. A bowhead whale does not have the intellect of reason, or the brilliance of mind. Turtles can live for hundreds of years. A specimen of the ocean quahog is recorded to be four hundred years old. Scientist has recorded some Antarctic Sponge to live to be more than a thousand years old. Numerous olive trees are well over 2,000 years old that are still alive today. The oldest tree in Europe is over 5,000 years old, and it is still alive.

If animals and trees can live for hundreds of years, then so can we. What is needed is the proper knowledge of how to eat to live abundantly.

**"Twenty years from now you will be more disappointed by the things that you didn't do than by the ones you did do, so throw off the bowlines, sail away from safe harbour, catch the trade winds in your sail. Explore, Dream, Discover."** – Mark Twain

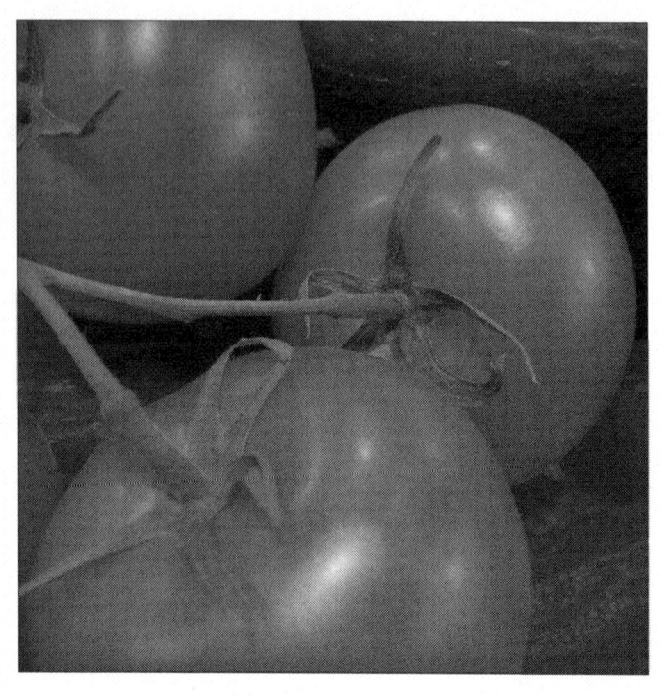

# CHAPTER 2
# Why one meal a day

## "Nothing is impossible, the word itself says 'I'm possible!'" – Audrey Hepburn

The more you use a thing, then the more you'll wear it out - if it's not given the proper rest and restoration. Here's a good example; to build the muscles, you will need to workout or put pressure on the muscles. But after the workout, the muscles will need proper rest. After working the muscles, you must rest so that the muscles can rebuild itself from the previous work. If you constantly work the muscles, you'll put strain on the muscles and ultimately damage yourself. The bodybuilders know this, so they only work each muscle group once every two or three days.

Eating three or six meals per day puts a lot of pressure on the stomach to digest the constant, excessive amount of food that we eat. Therefore, the body will use up a lot of its energy trying to digest the constant flow of food. After a time, the stomach gets worn out, which causes a multitude of problems.

Without the proper rest, and by eating six meals per day, the stomach won't have the time to properly digest the previous meal, so there's a build-up of toxins, and our system becomes polluted and weak. That is why one meal a day is the very best thing you could ever do (if you're currently eating three or six meals per day). The more rest you give your stomach, the more energy you'll have. For excessive food takes away energy from the body and makes us sluggish and lethargic.

In addition to the constant foods that we eat, some foods are really hard to digest, which puts double strain on our system. Foods like; nuts and meats are extremely hard to digest and may take a full 24 hours to digest, or even days.

That's the reason for the one meal a day concept. It gives the stomach proper rest to heal itself, and makes it strong and ready for the next meal.

This is the very best thing you could do for your health. It is even more important than the type of food that you decide to eat.

# CHAPTER 3
# The benefits of one meal a day

"The doctor of the future will give no medicines, but will interest his patients in the care of the human frame, in diet, and in the causes and prevention of diseases." – Thomas Edison

The amazing benefits of eating one meal per day are numerous and superlative. No other program can give you the type of benefits that comes from eating one meal per day (with the exception of one meal every two or three days).

**It cleanses the body of impurities and toxins.** Just about all foods contain small amounts of toxins and impurities, and over time, there's a build-up in our bodies (due to eating three and six meals per day). One meal per day flushes these toxins from our system.

**It gives you more abundant energy.** You'll have more energy as a result of you not wasting energy on digesting excessive foods.

**You will feel lighter and more agile.** This is a marvelous feeling.

**You will start looking younger.**

**Your skin will start to have a beautiful glow.** If you want smooth and soft skin with a natural, healthy glow, one meal per day will do it for you.

**Your eyes will become white and pure.** All the red, dull look of the eyes will vanish, and your eyes will begin to sparkle (like a new born child).

**Your mind becomes clearer.** The mind becomes more peaceful and calm.

**It saves you time and effort.** You don't have to be searching so often for food, or spending so much time preparing your food.

**It saves you money.** Eating six meals a day robs you of your health and your finances.

**It strengthens your will.** It can make you mentally stronger.

**It will cleanse the blood.**

**It shrinks the stomach.** This can help to reduce bloated stomach and belly fat.

**It makes you more alert** and will help you to become a quick thinker.

**It helps you to lose weight** if you're over-weight or obese. For the person who is obese, this is the very best and easiest way to lose weight (But for the person who wishes to maintain their body weight or to even gain a few pounds; read chapter 4).

**It makes you less acidic.**

**It helps to regulate your salt intake.** Most people unknowingly consume too much salt, but one meal a day helps to limit our salt intake.

**It slows the aging process** and can even reverse it. Depending on your level of commitment and dedication (along with a three day fast each month).

**It helps to remove pathogens** (fasting is effective against pathogens, and so is one meal a day).

**Sickness will begin to leave your body.** I've never seen a person who eats one meal a day (the right way) get sick.

**You'll be more resistant to the common cold and flu** (if practiced along with a monthly three day fast). The dedicated followers of the one meal a day program never gets the common cold or flu).

**It adds years to your life** (if practiced correctly, it can extend your life to 120 years or more).

**It makes you to feel better** (it's like a feel good tonic).

**It helps to regulate your sugar intake.**

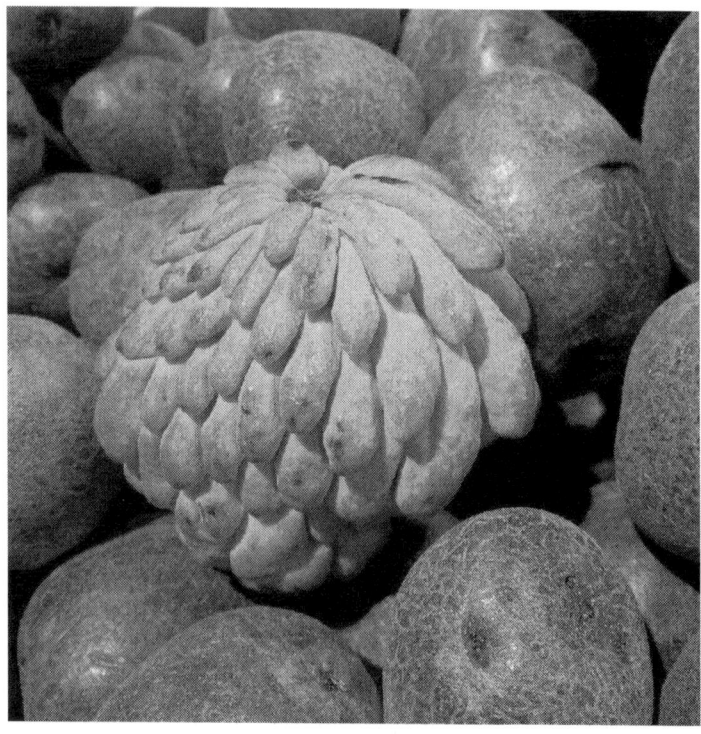

# CHAPTER 4

# Getting Started

"So many people spend their health gaining wealth, and then have to spend their wealth to regain their health." - A.J. Reb Materi

One meal a day is an amazingly simple program, but we all know that anything that has value carries a difficulty factor. This chapter will help you to master the one meal a day with very little difficulty. First and foremost, if you're currently eating between three and six meals a day, what I would first do is cut back to two meals a day for 21 days or until after the body gets used to the new routine, then I would slowly start practicing the one meal a day concept. This will help the body to gradually adjust to the new and better concept of one meal a day.

The first time that you try one meal a day, you will feel a bit hungry. It's not because you're hungry. No, it's because you've trained your stomach to eat at that particular time. So if you missed a meal, your stomach is just reminding you of the pattern that you have established over many years.

With each passing day, eating one meal a day becomes easier and easier, and within a short two weeks, you'll start to see that it is quite simple. After twenty one days of eating one meal a day (in the right way), you will begin to notice a major change. You won't feel hungry at all, and you will have more energy and vitality.

But remember; it is important to eat a big, nutritious meal every day. I'd find out how many calories needed for each day, and I make sure that I have it in my one meal.

The one meal a day concept is eating only one meal for the day, and nothing between meals.

However, it must be a healthy, nutritious meal. I eat one meal that is big enough to supply all my daily needs of calories, vitamins, minerals, proteins, carbohydrates, etc. And I slowly eat for two hours straight between the hours of 4pm – 6pm or 5pm – 7pm. I eat at the same time every day so that my stomach gets used to the new eating pattern.

The average person needs about 2,000 calories per day, depending on the level of activity. The person who don't eat the right amounts of calories each day will lose weight. To be successful at one meal per day, I regulate and monitor my calorie intake.

I try hard not to eat empty calories (foods that have been robbed of nutrients), that are found in white rice, white flour, white sugar, etc. Instead, I strive to eat whole wheat flour, which is much more delicious and nutritious than white flour. The very first time I tried to eat brown rice and whole wheat flour I thought it to be an acquired taste. But I was in for a pleasant surprise. It's all a matter of habit. Because I grew up eating white flour and white rice, I thought that whole wheat flour tasted "funny". Now I know the truth of it all; that white flour and white rice have very little flavor or taste, very little nutrients, and that whole wheat flour is supremely better and more delicious. Bottom line; it is best to eat foods that are wholesome and pure.

I never under-eat or over-eat, I just eat until I'm full. Eating fruits will cause you to feel full, but you will need more than just fruits and vegetables. Eat foods that will give good, slow burning energy. Navy beans give the body pure, clean, slow burning energy, or I find that organic brown rice or whole wheat flour gives good energy to last the entire day.

**NOTE:** One meal a day should only be practiced by adults that are 18 years old (or older). **For the person who aspires to lose weight, they can easily and rapidly lose weight by eating one meal a day. Just be sure to eat a healthy and nutritious meal and avoid eating so many calories while on the one meal a day program. This will surely eliminate obesity in a very short time. For the person who wants better and more rapid results; one meal every two days will give superlative results that are beyond your imagination, and will cause you to lose weight "overnight".**

**ADDITIONAL NOTE:** Here's the negative and positive of eating meat: **Meat is very hard to digest and it burdens the body, but it also gives strength. Eating a little meat every now and then will help you to keep your strength up. Beef is very good for strength** (especially for athletes, fighters and for hard, physical labour) and can make one meal a day that much easier. **But ultimately, it's best to eat lots of fruits and vegetables.**

One meal a day is an amazing concept that can give you stunning health and vitality. All it takes is for you to give it a chance and practice it for 21 days straight.

I've practiced the one meal per day concept for many years, and I'm here to tell you that it really works. It is the greatest thing you could do for your health, aside from eating one meal every two days.

Best wishes…

**"To keep the body in good health is a duty… otherwise we shall not be able to keep our mind strong and clear."** - Buddha

# BONUS SECTION

# Olive Oil Secrets

With so many new oils on the market today, and with all the increasingly negative health problems that people are starting to experience, I believe it is vitally necessary to shed some light on the topic.

It is imperative to know which oils to use in order to improve your health, and which oils to avoid in order for you to protect yourself from the extreme dangers that they pose.

Many people overlook the importance of choosing the right oil, thinking that it is a trivial matter. But in reality, it should be just as important as any other aspect of diet, for the type of oil you choose can turn your meal from a healthy one into one that is toxic and destructive to your health.

In addition to not knowing the right oil to choose, many people don't know the proper way of how to use oil. This is even more important than knowing the right oil to choose. If you choose the right oil, but use it in the wrong way, the end result would be negative.

The best thing to do is to choose the right oil and use it in the right way. This book will shed light on both paths so that you can increase your health and vitality.

## Fried foods

Admittedly, this may seem melodramatic, if not messianic. But it is quite possible you've never heard this before that oil is not to be used to fry your foods. No, not at all.

Let me explain.

**1.** Heating the oil will rapidly change the composition of the oil and kill some of the vital nutrients, thereby turning the oil from its pure state to making it slightly toxic and harder for the body to assimilate.

**2.** Foods that are fried are much more difficult and harder to digest, which is a major negative. If you care about your health and desire to be the very best version of you, then digestion is a critical aspect of health that must be looked at carefully. Foods that are hard to digest will burden the body over time and make it weak. Most people are oblivious to the fact that digestion is one of the most important aspects of health, and they fail to realize the two essential ways to properly evaluate food. The first way is to look at the nutritional value, and the second way is to look at how difficult it is to digest. Some foods are nutritious, but really hard to digest, which makes it unhealthy. The negative aspect of digestion would nullify the positive aspect of nutrition.

A good example would be peanuts, which are quite nutritious but extremely hard to digest, and in turn wears out the stomach and robs the unsuspecting individual of years, from just eating one meal of nuts. Eating nuts will take years off your life due to how difficult it is for the body to digest.

Fried food is very hard to digest and therefore should be completely avoided. So make sure that you only eat the very best foods that are easy for the body to digest.

## Proper use of oil

You can use your oil in many various ways; just make sure that it is not used for frying.

**In salads:** you can use your 100% extra virgin olive oil to lightly flavour your salad.

**In Soups:** your 100% extra virgin oil can be used to give your soup more nutrients and better flavour.

**In baking:** use good quality oil or butter for baking.

**As a dip:** use pure 100% extra virgin olive oil as a dip for your bread. Some oils are sweet and delicious, and will make your bread much tastier.

Be creative with your oil, there are many different ways to use it.

**Just remember to avoid using it to fry your food.**

## Olive oil

Olive oil has been used for thousands of years, and the olive trees are considered to be sacred in many places. Some olive trees live for thousands of years. Unlike canola oil, soya oil and corn oil which has been newly developed oils.

There are many varieties of olive oil on the market with varying quality. The very best is the 100% extra virgin olive oil that has been first cold pressed or cold extracted, using the most natural means of extraction. Some are processed and packaged the same day, while others may take days to bottle and processed, but generally speaking, the fresher the better. Olive oil is amazingly healthy and nutritious, and using it daily you'll start noticing how smooth and soft your skin will become in a very short time, believe you me, it's that good.

There are many different flavors to choose from. The connoisseurs of extra virgin olive oil knows this all too well. There are sweet, bittersweet, bitter, nutty, spicy, mild, to name a few. So therefore, you can choose the flavor that best suits your needs. It's sort of like wine; every vineyard has its own unique and distinctive taste.

This amazing oil cannot be compared to corn oil, for corn oil has the same consistent, bland flavor or the lack of it. It cannot be compared to canola oil, for canola oil is weak and flavorless. And it should not be compared to soya oil, for soya oil is cheaply produced oil. A matter of fact; corn, canola and soy are cheaply raised cattle food. They're not fit for human consumption

Olive oil is the very best oil there is. It has loads of monounsaturated fats, and it is very rich in antioxidants which help to strengthen the immune system to ward off viruses and various sicknesses.

Most of the olive oil on the market is not actually 100% extra virgin olive oil. Some olive oil that's labeled 100% extra virgin olive oil is not 100% pure. It's just a marketing trick used by commercializing people to deceive for the purpose of making more money. Some oils are mixed with other oils of lower quality. To avoid this, buy the oils that have been certified by one of the certification organizations to be 100% pure olive oil. Especially if you're going to spend a "pretty penny" on one of these oils, be sure to check the certification label. If there's no label, steer clear.

If you can't afford 100% extra virgin olive oil, regular olive oil is still better than most of the other oils on the market. So if you can't get the best of the best, make do with what you can afford for now. As things get better, you can gradually increase to the best of the best.

Olive oil is very sensitive to light, so avoid the ones in clear plastic or clear glass.

Try to get your 100% extra virgin olive oil in dark, glass bottles (the darker the better). Check the expiration date on the bottle and see when it was packaged, and be sure to use and store your oils properly. Once opened, be sure to use it within a month or two before it loses some of its natural goodness.

## Closing remarks

I know it's difficult to change the habits that we've developed over the years. But if we really want a change for the better in health and well-being, then we must strive hard to change the negative habits that robs us of health and vitality.

Be patient with yourself and gradually strive to change the negative habits into positive ones. I don't expect for you to change overnight, because I understand that many of us have been eating fried foods for decades. Therefore, it may take some time to break the habit, but strive to eliminate fried foods from your diet. You can do it.

If you want to have amazingly awesome health and long life, you can! The purpose of this book is to show you the right way to attain your desires. Now that you've seen the light, it is up to you to **walk therein.**

**"Let food be thy medicine and medicine be thy food."** - Hippocrates

# The Truth About Salt

I've researched the origins of salt to see when man started using this food substance, and to see if it was widely used by ancient civilizations.

It was intriguing to see very little information available, as if our ancient forefathers didn't use salt at all. The very first (widespread) use of salt as a food substance was by the Romans, which was considered to be a young (new) civilization at the time. Did the older and wiser civilizations use salt in their foods? Did they know of the extreme dangers and in turn, totally avoided salt?

Salt is a natural substance that is made up of sodium chloride, which is a mineral that is also found in many foods. Nature has already provided the perfect amount of salt in natural foods.

By adding more salt to foods, we end up masking the taste of the food while changing the natural composition of the food that nature intended. Nature intends for our food to have approximately 5% sodium or less, but when we add salt to our food it increases the sodium content of that food dramatically to 300%, 500%, 700% or even more, which in turn makes the food unnaturally toxic and unhealthy.

## How much salt?

If you must, consume no more than 1800 mg of salt each day (a teaspoon or less). It is extremely important for you to regulate your salt intake to the best of your ability.

The Canadian government says that more than 2,300 mg of salt is dangerous and recommends approximately 1,800 mg or less each day, but the majority of people consume more than 3,400 mg of salt every day, and many consume upwards of 6,000 mg per day.

This is where the extreme danger lies; **you not knowing the amount of salt you're consuming on a daily basis**. You could be ingesting upwards of 6,000 mg of salt each day and don't even know it, which can cause unnecessary suffering and serious damage to your health.

That is why you need to regulate your salt intake, so that you can stay within the safety limits.

Consume no more than 1,800 mg of salt each day. Measure and calculate the exact amount of salt that you consume each day. The inconvenience is a small price to pay for a longer and healthier life with increased beauty appearance. Excessive salt has a dulling and destructive effect on your beauty appearance. Regulating your salt intake will allow more of your natural beauty to shine through.

## Types of Salt

There are many types of salt on the market today, the very best salt is the pure, naturally moist sea salt. It has more minerals than the iodized white table salt and it is less potent and has more flavour. I use the Celtic Sea Salt of no more than 1,000 mg per day consistently, and I've never felt better. The more I cut back on my salt intake, the healthier I feel. Try to get the salt that has been certified kosher. This certification gives an added layer of security.

Regardless of how pure the salt is, it is still extremely dangerous. The point here is that excessive salt is not necessary for our bodies (sodium chloride is necessary, not salt). Yes, it is good for flavouring foods, but it is neither good nor necessary for health.

The iodized white table salt is the worst kind of salt you can ever consume. It is even more dangerous than the regular pure sea salt. I would suggest that you try to avoid this salt completely. For just a few cents more, you can upgrade to the pure, natural, kosher sea salt.

## Ideas to limit your salt intake

Limiting your salt intake can be quite easy if you have proper guidance.

### Here are a few tips on how to limit your salt intake:

1. **Eat lots of vegetables**; you don't have to add salt to vegetables and they will taste just as delicious without the salt and you won't even notice that there's no salt.

2. **Instead of salty snacks**; eat more natural fruits that are loaded with vitamins, minerals and antioxidants.

3. **Avoid processed foods**; processed foods are loaded with salt in order to mask the inadequate taste and to extend the shelf life. Furthermore, extra salt is added to get more people hooked.

4. **Avoid the salt shaker**; you don't need this, it encourages negative habits.

5. **Stay away from restaurants**; they add loads of salt to their foods. Plus, you'll need to regulate you salt intake and restaurants makes it extremely difficult to do this, for most restaurants won't tell you the amount of salt that is contained in their meals. A few fast food restaurants will tell you the salt content of each meal. But generally speaking, they don't. And if they do, the salt content is usually very high, so steer clear.

6. **Use pure, naturally moist sea salt**; this type of salt is less potent. It is less destructive and it has more minerals.

7. **Cook your rice without salt**; then eat with gravy or meat that was lightly flavoured with salt.

8. **Use more spices and herbs to flavour your foods**; this will help you to cut back on the amount of salt that you use.

9. **Drink less artificial juices**; some artificial sodas and juices contains salt, look out!

10. **Drink more water**; this helps to flush the excessive salt from your body.

11. Best of all, be diligent and focused; it is easy to lose focus and get distracted, so strive to stay on the path.

Most product labels will only give sodium information instead of salt. Sodium is just a part of salt so it is important not to get the two confused. 1 gram of sodium = 2.5 grams of salt.

# Closing remarks

Salt is like a slow poison. Using salt for just a few days will not cause any major harm, but using so much of it consistently for years will surely hurt us. It will take years to do damage to the human body. Therefore, the earlier you learn to regulate your salt intake, the better. I've been using salt for many years, but now I see the clear and present dangers and now I eat less than 1,800 mg each day.

It takes 21 days to get used to eating without excessive salt, and once you pass the 21 days, you won't even miss the salt and your food will taste amazingly delicious.

Teach your children about the dangers of salt. Give them friendly reminders as to the extreme dangers and help them to build healthy habits from a young age so that it will be easier for them later in life. The reason why we're so hooked on salt is because from a very young age we established negative salty habits. If you want the absolute best for your children, never allow your child to get hooked on salty foods, it can become a life-long habit that can eventually cause premature health problems.

I can think of no other substance that is as dangerous as salt. It is by far the most dangerous substance that we consume. Why is it so dangerous? Because we eat so much of it and it then accumulates in our bodies. The average person consumes salt three to six times per day with breakfast, lunch and dinner. This makes it hard for our bodies to eliminate the constant intake of salt.

I would recommend that you do all in your power to regulate your salt intake. Do it for the sake of life, health, family, and beauty.

You deserve the best.

And best of all, stay positive.

# Supreme health

What do you think is the most precious thing to own on the planet? Is it a billion dollars? Is it a truck full of diamonds? Is it a lavishly appointed Bugatti Vincero? Emphatically no! It is you. You're the most precious thing in the universe. More precious than the sun, moon and stars combine. But yet, most of us would take better care of a Bugatti or Ferrari than we would of ourselves. We would feed those cars supreme fuel, yet we eat the worst and cheapest foods.

If death knocks on our door, we would give it all up in an instant, just to hold on to our precious life - which shows clearly that your life and health is vastly more important than anything else. Then why be nonchalant about it. Why not take great care of yourself since you're the most precious creation in the universe.

# What to Eat

Eat nothing but the purest and healthiest foods, and eat lots of fruits and vegetables.

Broccoli is one of the healthiest vegetable around. It has lots of antioxidants and vitamins, and it is easy to cook and easy to digest. Then there's asparagus, cauliflower, zucchini, etc.

You can eat as much onions and garlic as you like, for they are supremely healthy. Almost all fruits and vegetables are good for you, with the exception of a few that are listed in part two of this book. Navy beans are also supremely healthy; if you want amazing energy, eat lots of navy beans. Just soak the beans overnight to remove the excess gas.

Organic brown rice is also good; just make sure that you rinse it many times to remove the excess starch. Whole wheat flour is also good, and whole wheat bread is excellent; just make sure you toast it, so it won't rise again in your stomach.

Fish is very healthy. Try your best to eat fresh wild fish, and avoid the farmed ones. Make sure the fish weights no more than ten pounds, the smaller the fish, the better. The larger species of fish tend to have more pollution and toxins stored in their bodies.

Use spices to add flavor and nutrients to your meals, try using natural fresh spices and avoid the dried-up stuff on the supermarket shelves.

Onions and garlic are supremely well crafted - they have layers and layers of protection, they have healing properties and they are supremely nutritious. Raw garlic and onions are potent and powerful, so be careful and steam them well (lightly steamed). They'll add an avalanche of flavors and nutrients to your meal.

## "Personal beauty is a greater recommendation than any letter of reference." - Aristotle

### How to properly eat

Eat only one meal per day (adults 18 and over). This is by far the best thing you could do for your health. This is the secret that the ancient people used in order to live a very long time. Eating three meals per day stresses the body, which is why the modern man lives only a short life, because he eats too often.

## What to Drink

Drink pure spring water. It is the very best type of water. A normal healthy person can get by with just one glass of water per day, but considering that most people are dehydrated and acidic nowadays, it is recommended to drink eight glasses each day.

Drink lots of pure, clean wholesome milk. It is so healthy that a person could live off milk exclusively for a very long time. What makes it so good? Well, it is loaded with nutrients, and it is very easy to digest (foods that are hard to digest stresses the body and causes pre-mature aging and sickness).

Drink pure and natural fruit juices (freshly squeezed).

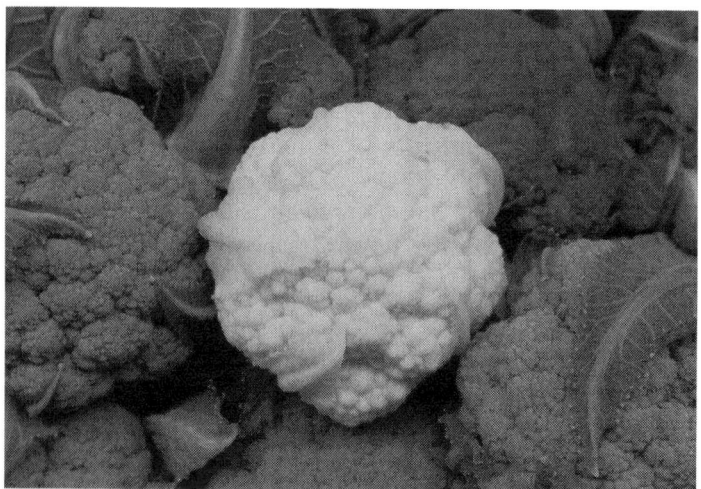

# Closing remarks

It all boils down to habit. If for 30 days of the month you eat all junk foods, or processed foods; then for one day you decide to eat the healthiest and the best foods known to man, the overall result that you get will be a negative one. Because for 30 days you've been doing all negatives, so the one day of positive is not enough.

On the other hand, if you eat nothing but the purest and most wholesome foods for 30 days, then one day you decide to go out and eat all the greasy, fatty, salty, starchy foods you can find; the overall result you get for the month would be a very positive one. The one day of negative is not enough to nullify the positives that you've been doing for the 30 consecutive days.

Supreme health comes from what you do consistently, not what you do occasionally. Therefore, try to be diligent in consistently eating the right foods and at the right time.

*Live your Life*

## ABOUT THE AUTHOR

Author Jason Antonio Drysdale is an aspiring wordsmith, covering the vital and immense topics of health and wealth. His hobbies include yachting and flying. He's also a connoisseur of the finer things in life.

Printed in Great Britain
by Amazon